FLAT BELLY DIET
ZERO FLAT FROM YOUR BELLY

Lara Weil

Disclaimer

While all attempts have been made to verify the information provided in this book, the author doesn't assume any responsibility for errors, omissions, or contrary interpretations of the subject matter contained within. The information provided in this book is for educational and entertainment purposes only. The reader is responsible for his or her own actions and the author does not accept any responsibilities for any liabilities or damages, real or perceived, resulting from the use of this information.

The trademarks that are used are without any consent, and the publication of the trademark is without permission or backing by the trademark owner. All trademarks and brands within this book are for clarifying purposes only and are the owned by the owners themselves, not affiliated with this document.

Contents

Book Description

This book asserts that certain foods cut off fat qualities, turning off the parts of our DNA that trigger weight pick up and enacting our bodies to blaze, not store, fat. It says that consuming the right eating regimen can basically take your foot off the fat-quality quickening agent and drastically turn around weight increase, in the process actually changing your hereditary predetermination. It contends that fitting assimilation controls aggravation, a frequently neglected guilty party in weight addition, and that certain foods make provocative reactions in numerous individuals. It claims to turn off your fat-stockpiling qualities by concentrating on nine force nutrition classes that are connected specifically to the developing study of healthful hereditary qualities. You can get the breakfast and dinner recipes which will help you to do diet. Simply download this book and make your cooking agreeable and charming.

Introduction

The 'Flat Belly' eating regimen is said to "turn off" or die down the qualities that cause corpulence while being sound in the meantime. Food items such as beans, almond and oats within this ingesting program are said to evacuate your gut microscopic organisms, contributing to annihilating your characteristics that cause Diabetes.

"Instinctive Fat" is a kind of fat that adds to a fatty gut, and Chorine in which emanates from consuming eggs, destroys in which; this is something the system supports incorporating in the gut cutter's eating routine.

Utilizing Olive Oil as a part of the dietary calendar controls the health food nuts' long for delayed hours that aides in containing the amount of is consumed consistently. With all these good dieting propensities in actuality, the tummy fat is said to diminishing without a doubt.

Zinczenko states his eating regimen arrangement is a direct consequence of his individual encounters in life as a hefty child and his father, who most likely kicked the bucket of corpulence as well. This individual indicated in the awaken of utilizing the software that the standard one that employs the dict program arrangement will lose close to some ins of instinct in the moment of six to eight weeks.

The idea in the arrangement is usually to halt phenomena such as bloating, that are fundamental in individuals with temperamental degrees of obliged food, hence disposing of the actual qualities that retailer excess fat systems.

Acknowledging what stomach fat can do, and what it prompts is vital. Ailments that accompany being corpulent incorporate heart strokes, sort 2 diabetes and hypertension, to give some examples, and with Zinczenko's "Flat Belly" eating routine, embracing a sound way of life and physical activity has been prescribed by wellbeing specialists to accomplish the obliged results.

Chapter 1: Step by step instructions to drop Belly Fat with the Flat Belly Diet

Pregame lunch and dinner with greens

Verdant greens like collard greens, kale, watercress, and arugula may not be on your ordinary rundown, nevertheless each and every one surround a composite called sulforaphane. This supplement has been demonstrated to act straightforwardly on the qualities.

A healthier admission of the compound means a healthier body weight for you. Furthermore, only a meager teaspoon of vinaigrette will help your body assimilate the fat-dissolvable supplements

Swap farmed salmon for wild salmon

Incline protein like fish is an extraordinary approach to battle fat and support your digestion system. Yet the salmon you get at the nearby market may not be the best wagered for your belly. The cold water fish has a merited disrepute for pressing a lot of heart-solid omega 3 fatty acids—1,253 mg of the well done, and only 114 mg of provocative, stomach busting omega 6s.

Yet the cultivated assortment and 90 percent of what we consume today is cultivated has an altogether different story to tell. It packs an incredible 1,900 mg of unfortunate omega-6s.

Have dark chocolate & berries for dessert

Savoring delightful nourishment is a fundamental principle of the Flat Belly Diet. The balanced, "zero sacrifice" approach played a crucial role in assisting test panelist Jennie Joshi in shedding her post-pregnancy weight. Within just over a month on the Flat Belly Diet, Jennie shed 11 pounds, declaring, "and the post-pregnancy bulge is disappearing!" she exclaimed. "I couldn't believe I was indulging in dark chocolate—and finally seeing results! It's a lifestyle, not a diet. It's easy to stick to, and it makes sense."

Rethink Your Supplements

In case you're taking heaps of vitamins and robotics every day, you may need to reexamine your technique. Expanded levels of B vitamins have long been connected with a higher predominance of stoutness and diabetes, maybe in light of the fact that mega dosing triggers our fat qualities.

An everyday multivitamin is likely fine; yet don't attempt to persuade yourself that more is better. Furthermore, a late study by ConsumerLab.com found that most business probiotics have far fewer solid microbes than they assert. Your better wager is to concentrate on the Flat Belly sustenance's to guarantee your gut is getting a lot of adoration and your fat qualities are being cut off at the pass.

Eat a Better Peanut Butter

Genuine nutty spread is made with two fixings: peanuts, and possibly some salt. You realize that peanuts issue you gut thinning monounsaturated fats, tummy-filling fiber, and protein, which boosts digestion system.

But be watchful of the brand you purchase: in the event that you see fixings like sugar, palm oil, or anything you can't contend, deposit it reverses. They will challenge any immense the peanuts may do.

Unexercised

The most compelling motivation we can't stick to our workouts? No time. Attempting to crush a trek to the rec center, with a shower and change of garments, into a boisterous calendar predominantly around the occasions can make even the most committed wellness buff into somebody, well, less buff.

Yet researchers in New Zealand as of late found that men and ladies who occupied with three 10-moment exercise "appetizers" before breakfast, lunch and dinner saw brought down blood glucose levels—a fat-busting advantage these people demonstrated throughout the day!

Make Your Own Trail Mix

The three noteworthy fixings of an impeccable Flat Belly dinner or nibble are protein, fiber and sound fats, and each of the three can be found in wealth in a decent trail blend.

Tragically, most business blends are made with additional oils, salt, and sugar. Stir up your own particular from a determination of nuts, seeds, unsweetened dried organic product, and dim chocolate pieces. Make a point to incorporate peanuts: they're a top wellspring of both genistein and resveratrol, two supplements that help lessen the activity of your fat-stockpiling qualities.

Mix Up a Magic Elixir

Begin every day by making a substantial pitcher of "spa water"—that is water loaded with cut entire lemons, oranges or grapefruits—and make a state of tasting some way or another through no less than 8 glasses before time to beat the silage.

Citrus untreated goods are affluent in the cancer prevention agent DE limonene, a capable compound found in the peel that invigorates liver proteins to help flush poisons from the body and gives lazy guts a kick.

Power Up With Eggs

You'll discover lean, satisfying protein in each and every chomp you tackle Flat Belly Diet. The muscle-building nutrient is crucial for the arrangement, and eggs happen to be one of the most effortless and most adaptable conveyance frameworks in the universe.

Not just that, they're additionally the most obvious dietary wellspring of a supplement called choline. Choline, which is discovered likewise in lean meats, fish and collard greens, assaults the quality component that triggers your body to store fat around your liver.

One Flat Belly Diet formula a breakfast hash with sweet potatoes and new homestead eggs—got to be test panelist Morgan Minor's go-to breakfast, and after only 3 weeks on the system, the female firefighter lost 11 pounds and 4 inches from her waist!

Stir up a plant- protein smoothie

Protein beverages are incredible approaches to get beast measurements of gut busting sustenance into a basic nibble. Most commercial beverages are loaded with unpronounceable chemicals that can agitate our gut wellbeing and reason aggravation and bloat.

Furthermore, the high dosages of whey used to help protein levels can increase the gut bloating impact. The Flat Belly arrangement: Try vegetarian protein, which has the same fat-blazing and muscle-building advantages, without the bloat.

Make Some Guacamole

For test panelist June Caron, consolidating new deliver like avocados was an extraordinary lesson from Flat Belly diet. The 55 year-old vanished 6 pounds in the earliest week on the mission. I am never eager. What's more the weight simply keeps on slipping away! Sound nails, glowing skin, along with superior sleep were Flat Belly rewards.

Pick Red Fruit Over Green

It's the best organic product for weight reduction. The larger amounts of supplements called flavonoids—especially anthocyanins, exacerbates that give red organic products their shading smooth the activity of fat-stockpiling qualities. Indeed, red-bellied stone organic products like plums brag phenolic aggravates that have been indicated to regulate the statement of fat qualities.

Chapter 2 – The Best Zero-Belly Superfoods

Flat Belly lives up to expectations in three routes: by decreasing bloat, recuperating your gut and turbo charging your digestion system. These three instruments work in coupled to turn off your fat qualities resetting your body to "slim."

The key is to rebalance you're eating regimen with the Flat Belly sustenance's. This 9 sustenance's are similar to delightful little IT prodigies, hacking into your body's PC framework and resetting your hereditary code to "thin."

Z: FLAT BELLY Drinks. These are smoothies that are supercharged with paunch straightening supplements. The key: every beverage is stuffed with protein, solid fats and fiber. Here's a brisk formula I call the Mango Muscle-Up: Mix 1 scoop veggie lover protein powder, ⅔ glass solidified mango lumps, ½ tbsp almond margarine, ½ container unsweetened almond and coconut milk. You'll receive up to 29 grams of proteins for just 224 calories from fat.

E: Eggs. Eggs are the most obvious wellspring of choline, a fat-blazing supplement. They start up your digestion system and they help turn off the qualities for stomach fat stockpiling.

R: Red Fruits. Why red? They pack the most phytonutrients—high-fueled exacerbates that make your tummy fat see red.

O: Olive Oil and Other Healthy Fats. Sound fats compel your body to smolder calories all the more productively. Don't stress: consuming fat won't make you fat any more than consuming cash will make you rich. Talking about sound consumes, get your level tummy fix with the fundamental 8 Foods That Beat the Bloat.

B: Beans and Other Healthy Fiber. You have 80 trillion organisms in your stomach, and the vast majority of them are furious. Solid fiber is the thing that we call "prebiotic," significance it nourishes the sound microbes and helps them battle aggravation and fat addition.

E: Extra Plant Protein. I add protein to the FLAT BELLY Drinks to help support digestion system. However, most protein is produced using whey, which can prompt bloating. That is the reason I utilize plant protein. This arrangement diminishes bloating drastically up to 3 inches off your waistline in the first week.

L: Lean Meat and Fish. Protein is kryptonite to tummy fat. I need you to consume steak, shrimp—even burgers!

L: Leafy Greens and Brightly Colored Vegetables. Verdant greens issue you folate, which prevents fat-cell arrangement.

Y: Your Favorite Spices: ginger, cinnamon and even dim chocolate. Why chocolate? Your solid gut loves it!

Chapter 3: Flat Belly Fat Breakfast Recipes

Banana Pancakes with Walnut Honey

Prep time: 15 minutes
Cook time: 15 minutes
Makes: 4 servings

Ingredients:
Hotcakes
1⅓ c Easy Pancake Mix* or locally acquired, trans-fat free hotcake blend
¼ tsp ground cinnamon
1 c low-fat buttermilk
¼ c water
1 egg
1 Tbsp canola oil
1 tsp vanilla concentrate
1 lg banana, divided the long way and cut dainty cuts
½ c crisp raspberries
Walnut Honey
½ c walnuts, cleaved (MUFA)
⅓c nectar
1 Tbsp water

Directions:
1. Consolidate the flapjack blend and cinnamon in a substantial dish. Consolidate the buttermilk, water, egg, oil, and vanilla concentrate in a different dish. Race into the flapjack blend and mix until smooth. Overlay in the banana. Put aside.

2. Join the walnuts, nectar, and water in a little bowl.

3. Cover an expansive nonstick skillet with cooking shower and set over medium warmth. Include the flapjack player in sparse ¼ cupfuls and cook, in groups, for around 2 minutes or until the hotcakes have puffed and the undersides are daintily seared. Turn the flapjacks and cook for around 2 minutes longer or until daintily carmelized. Present with the walnut nectar and raspberries.

Nutrition facts per serving:
425 cal, 10 g ace, 67 g carb, 15 g fat, 2 g sat fat, 55 mg chol, 387 mg sodium, 5 g fiber.

Tropical Fruit Smoothie

Prep time: 2.5 minutes
Cook time: 2.5 minutes
Makes: 2 servings

Ingredients:
1½ c solidified mango solid shapes or peach cuts, somewhat defrosted, or 1 lg mango, peeled and cut off pit
1 c hulled, divided new strawberries
1 c without fat vanilla yogurt or light vanilla soy milk
½ c chilled mango nectar
1 Tbsp solidified pineapple juice condensed, marginally defrosted
2 Tbsp flaxseed oil (MUFA)

Directions:
1. Place mango, strawberries, yogurt, nectar, and juice condensed in blender. On the off chance that utilizing new mango, include 4 or 5 ice 3D shapes. Mix until decently consolidated and smooth.

Add oil and mix just to consolidate. Pour into 2 glasses. Topping every glass with a strawberry on the off chance that you have additional items.

Nutrition facts every serving:

400 cal, 65 g carb, 15 g fat, 5 g fiber, 86 mg sodium, 2 mg chol, 1.5 g sat fat, 8 g expert,
 Huevos Rancheros

Prep time: 15 minutes
Cook time: 15 minutes
Makes: 4 servings

Ingredients:
1 tsp ground cumin
1 can (15 oz) no-salt included pink beans, flushed and depleted
4 scallions, cut
1 sm red ringer pepper, cut into meager strips
½ c diminished sodium chicken juices
2 cloves garlic, minced
4 eggs
1 c cut avocado (MUFA)
4 Tbsp without fat Greek-style yogurt
4 Tbsp salsa
8 (6") corn tortillas, toasted
Dash of hot-pepper sauce

Directions:
HEAT a 10" nonstick skillet over medium-high warmth. Include the cumin and cook, blending once in a while, for around 30 seconds or until fragrant. Include the beans, scallions, chime pepper, soup, and garlic.

Heat to the point of boiling, then lessen the warmth so the mixture stews. Cook for 8 minutes or until the vegetables are delicate and the vast majority of the stock is vanished. With the back of a huge silicone or wooden spoon, crush the beans until they are knotty.

2. Utilize the back of the spoon to make 4 spaces in the beans. Working each one in turn, break every egg into a custard glass and pour in every space. Cover and cook for around 8 minutes or until the eggs are cooked to the coveted doneness.

3. Scoop every share of egg-topped bean mixture onto a plate. Scramble the avocado cuts over and around the beans. Top every presenting with 1 Tbsp of the yogurt and 1Tbsp of the salsa. Present with the tortillas and hot-pepper sauce, if sought.

Nutrition facts every serving:
331 cal, 16 g master, 42 g carb, 12 g fat, 3 g sat fat, 250 mg sodium, 10 g fiber, 1 mg cholesterol
Eggs Florentine with Sun-Dried Tomato Pesto

Prep time: 15 minutes
Cook time: 15 minutes
Makes: 4 servings

Ingredients:
1 tsp olive oil
1 bundle (9 oz) prewashed spinach
⅓cwithout fat Greek-style yogurt
¼ c sun-dried tomato pesto (MUFA)
1 tsp vinegar
Squeeze of salt
4 huge eggs
2 entire grain English biscuits, part and toasted
Newly ground dark pepper

Directions:
1. HEAT the oil in a huge nonstick skillet over medium-high warmth. Include the spinach and cook (in clumps, if essential) until shriveled.

2. Consolidate the yogurt and pesto. Blend ¼ c into the spinach and expel from the warmth. Spread to keep warm.

3. In the meantime, warm a medium pot containing 1" of water to a bubble over high warmth. Include the vinegar and salt and diminish the warmth to low. Break an egg into a custard mug and tenderly tip the egg into the water. Rehash with the staying 3 eggs. Cover and stew, shaking the skillet for 3 minutes for a delicate cooked yolk or until the whites are totally situated and the yolks start to thicken.

4. PLACE an English biscuit half on each of 4 warm plates. Spoon the spinach onto every biscuit. Evacuate the eggs with an opened spoon, and deplete over paper towels (still in the spoon), before setting on the spinach.

5. Blend 1 Tbsp of the poaching fluid into the yogurt mixture to make it smoother. Spoon equally over every egg and crush some pepper absurd.

Nutrition facts every serving:
175 cal, 21.1 g carb, 6.1 g fat, 2 g sat fat, 450 mg sodium, 200 mg cholesterol, 12 g expert, 5 g fiber
Cranberry-Pecan Scones

Prep time: 20 minutes
Cook time: 20 minutes
Makes: 8 servings

Ingredients:
2 c entire wheat baked good flour
1 c pecans, slashed (MUFA)
2 tsp preparing powder
½ tsp preparing pop
½ tsp salt
1¼ c low-fat vanilla yogurt
2 Tbsp canola oil
1 tsp newly ground orange get-up-and-go
⅔ c dried sweetened cranberries

Directions:

1. PREHEAT the stove to 400°F. Delicately layer a 9" round heating container with cooking shower.

2. WHISK together the flour, pecans, preparing powder, heating pop, and salt in an extensive dish.

3. WHISK together the yogurt, oil, and orange get-up-and-go in a little bowl.

4. MAKE a well in the core of the flour mixture and include the yogurt mixture and cranberries. Mix just until mixed.

5. PRESS into the arranged dish. Score the batter with a blade to structure 8 triangles. Prepare for 20 to 25 minutes or until gently cooked and a wooden toothpick embedded in the inside confesses all out.

Nutrition facts every serving:
308 cal, 6 g genius, 38 g carb, 15 g fat, 1.5 g sat fat, 2 mg chol, 350 mg sodium, 5 g fiber.

Chapter 4: Flat Belly Fat Lunch & Dinner Recipes

Steak-and-Pepper Tacos

Prep time: 20 minutes
Cook time: 25 minutes
Makes: 4 servings

Ingredients:
1 pound flank or peg steak
Juice of 1 lime, in addition to lime wedges for serving
1 teaspoon genuine salt
2 garlic cloves, pounded
1/2 teaspoon mellow stew powder
3 teaspoons vegetable oil
1/2 red onion, cut
3 chime peppers, 1 every red, yellow, and orange, daintily cut
1/2 container new or solidified corn pieces
8 little corn tortillas, warmed
1/2 avocado, cut
1/4 container ground low-fat Monterey Jack
1/4 container salsa verde or 2 tablespoons hacked new cilantro
2 tablespoons cut cured jalapenos
Decreased fat sharp cream (discretionary)

Directions:
1. Marinate the steak in the lime juice, salt, garlic, and stew powder in a fixed plastic sack for 20 to 30 minutes.

2. Then, warm a substantial cast-iron skillet over high warmth for 5 minutes. Include 2 teaspoons of the vegetable oil to the skillet. Include the red onion and ringer peppers; cook, throwing much of the time, for 5 minutes. Add the corn and keep on cooking until the peppers are singed and delicate, around 3 more minutes. Exchange the vegetables to a dish and keep warm.

3. Wipe the skillet with a paper towel and warmth for an alternate moment. Include the remaining teaspoon of vegetable oil. Take the steak from the marinade, then dry with paper towels. Place the steak in the skillet, diminish warmth to medium-high, cook 7-10 minutes, turning once half of the way finished. Exchange to a board and let rest for 5 minutes.

4. Cut the steak over the grain and organize on a platter with all the peppers along with limescale wedges. Make tacos with all the comfy tortillas, avocado, Monterey Jack port, salsa, jalapenos along with, in the event that searched for, sharpened cream.

Nutrition facts every serving:
416 calories, 32g protein, 38g carbohydrate, 16g fat (4.3g immersed), 7g fiber.

Lemon-Walnut Chicken

Prep time: 10 minutes
Cook time: 10 minutes
Makes: 4 servings

Ingredients:
2 tablespoons finely slashed parsley*
2 tablespoons finely slashed toasted walnuts*
1/4 teaspoon finely ground lemon pizzazz
4 medium skinless, boneless chicken breast parts, beat to 1/2-inch thickness
2 teaspoons universally handy flour
1/2 teaspoon salt
1/2 teaspoon dark pepper
1 tablespoon olive oil
3 tablespoons diced shallots
1/4 glass low-sodium chicken stock
1 tablespoon crisp lemon juice, in addition to lemon wedges for serving
1/4 glasses chestnut basmati rice, steamed

Directions:
1. In a little bowl, combine the parsley, walnuts, and lemon pizzazz. Dust the chicken with the flour and season with the salt and dark pepper.

2. In an extensive skillet (or two medium-huge skillets), warm the olive oil over medium warmth. Include the shallots and saute until they start to turn translucent, 1 moment. Push the shallots to the other side of the dish, include the chicken bosoms, and cook until brilliant, around 2 minutes every side.

3. Pour the chicken soup and lemon juice into the dish. Protect, and also enable stew around low friendliness before state of mind run clear once the chicken can be pierced, 3 to 4 far more minutes.

4. Use tongs to exchange the chicken to a serving dish, leaving the fluid and shallots in the container. Heat the fluid to the point of boiling over medium warmth and blend until thickened, 1 moment. Merge the actual parsley blend. Put the actual spices within the fowl and assist within the rice with all the fruit wedges.

Nutrition facts every serving:
calories, 36g protein, 19g carbohydrate, 8g fat (1.3g immersed), 2g fiber.

Shrimp-and-Avocado Rice Bowl

Prep time: 10 minutes
Cook time: 10 minutes
Makes: 4 servings

Ingredients:
16 medium cleaned, shelled, tail-on shrimp (around 3/4 pound), defrosted if solidified
2 teaspoons sesame oil

1/2 teaspoons nectar
Little squeeze cayenne pepper
2 eggs, delicately beaten
1 tablespoon light soy sauce
1 tablespoon rice wine vinegar
1 container shelled edamame, steamed
2 teaspoons toasted sesame seeds
1/4 containers short-grain cocoa rice, cooked by directions
1 ready avocado, cut

Directions:
1. Preheat the oven. In a medium ovenproof container, throw the shrimp with 1 teaspoon each of the sesame oil and the nectar. Add the cayenne.

2. Lay the shrimp level. Cook for 2 minutes every side.

3. Warmth just a little nonstick griddle over medium heat and can include the residual teaspoon of sesame gas. Dump inside ovum. Prepare food undisturbed right up until collection, around 3 units. Flip and cook until simply set on the second side, 1 more moment. Exchange to a board and cut into strips.

4. In a little bowl, consolidate the soy sauce and rice wine vinegar with the staying 1/2 teaspoon nectar.

5. Fold the edamame and sesame seeds into the rice. Function the particular rice in dishes finished with all the egg pieces, shrimp, in addition to avocado. Area the particular soy-vinegar combination inside a tiny pan in addition to utilization for the kitchen table for showering.

Nutrition facts every serving:
calories, 30g protein, 56g carbohydrate, 16g fat (2.8g immersed), 6g fiber.

Spinach-Mushroom Pizza

Prep time: 20 minutes
Cook time: 15 minutes
Makes: 6 servings

Ingredients:
1 12-ounce entire wheat pizza outside, for example, Boboli
1/4 mug pizza sauce
1/2 mug solidified spinach, defrosted and depleted well
1/4 little red onion, daintily cut
1 mug destroyed part-skim mozzarella
6 medium cremini mushrooms, cut
1/4 mug part-skim ricotta
2 tablespoons ground Parmesan
1 tablespoon virgin olive oil
2 teaspoons balsamic vinegar

Directions:
1. Preheat the stove to 450 degrees. Place an extensive substantial heating sheet on the base of the stove. Lay the pizza outside layer on a work surface.

2. Distribute the surface level while using the marinade, had taken soon after with the spinach in addition to onion. Dust while using the mozzarella in addition to mushrooms. Touch the ricotta over the pizza and sprinkle with the Parmesan. Shower the olive oil everywhere.

3. Utilize a meager curtailing of a second preparing sheet to deliberately exchange the pizza to the preheated heating sheet on the base of the broiler. Heat until the outside is puffed and starting to shading at the edges and the cheddar is dissolved, 10 minutes. Take the sheet out of the stove and preheat the oven.

4. Cook the pizza, observing deliberately, until the cheddar is cooked and rising, around 2 minutes. Let pizza cool on the sheet for 5 minutes. Mix with all the balsamic vinegar, reduce in to wedges, as well as provide.

Nutrition facts every serving:
252 calories, 15g protein, 30g carbohydrate, 10g fat (3.5g immersed), 5g fiber.

Cumin Salmon with Yogurt-Cucumber Sauce

Prep time: 15 minutes
Cook time: 10 minutes
Makes: 4 servings

Ingredients:
2 teaspoons virgin olive oil
1/2 teaspoon ground cumin
1/2 teaspoon sugar
1/2 teaspoon dark pepper
1/2 teaspoon salt, in addition to a squeeze
4 salmon filets (around 4 ounces each)
1/2 container nonfat Greek yogurt
1 huge pickling diced cucumber
1 scallion, trimmed and finely hacked
3 tablespoons minced new parsley
1 teaspoon new lemon juice
8 ounces entire wheat orzo, cooked by directions

Directions:
1. In a dish, consolidate the olive oil, cumin, sugar, dark pepper, and 1/2 teaspoon salt. Lay the salmon on a foil-lined heating sheet and brush the finish with the oil mixture. Cool for appr. 15 minutes.

2. Preheat the oven. Join the yogurt, cucumber, scallion, parsley, lemon juice, and the remaining squeeze of salt in a little bowl.

3. Cook the salmon until it is scarcely obscure at the inside of the thickest section, 7 to 10 minutes. Serve over the orzo, finished with the yogurt sauce.

Nutrition facts every serving:

487 calories, 34g protein, 45g carbohydrate, 19g fat (3.8g immersed), 10gfiber.

Chapter 5: Unusual Tips and Foods That Boost Fat Loss

On the off chance that you need to drop fat quick, never go to rest without consuming a Slim Jim. Ok. Perhaps you shouldn't pick a slim jim however you can drop fat 32% speedier if, as opposed to going to couch ravenous like the vast majority used to think, you have a little plate of protein.

Chill to shed those last few pounds of fat. Individuals who shower in cool to frosty water smolder, overall, 100 additional calories amid their shower than the individuals who absorb a hot shower.

Frosty water compels your body to work extra time to keep up its typical temperature! Consider off. The individuals who figure out how to stay asleep for the entire evening smolder fat 2 times more efficiently than individuals who thrash around, or get up frequently amid the night.

Figure out how to spit. In the event that you get a support from sugary beverages amid your workout, you're not the only one! Games beverages issue us a support in 2 courses (by issuing us a little sugar-high, yet similarly as fortifying to your framework is the mental help you get from the taste of the sugary beverage).

So on the off chance that you truly need to be incline, you have to figure out how to spit. By taking a sizable chunk of a games beverage like Gatorade and spitting it out, you'll get the mental support in vitality you require without the sugar that makes fat stick to your body.

Never consume before the TV. Individuals who consume before the TV, by and large, consume 29% more nourishment. Furthermore, a recent report by Yale University demonstrated that individuals who viewed sustenance related advertisements consumed 45% more!

Conclusion

Flat Belly Diet demonstrates to you proper methodologies to deactivate your fat qualities, rev up your digestion system, expatriate bloat, and equalization your digestive wellbeing, permitting you to effortlessly fabricate incline, solid stomach muscle and strip away undesirable paunch fat without relinquishing calories or investing hours at the rec center. The outcome: weight reduction that is less demanding, quicker, all the more enduring, and tastier than you'd ever envision.

Any eating routine arrangement can guarantee you weight reduction. What Flat Belly offers you is something more: the ability to wield sustenance as a weapon, to turn off your fat qualities, support your digestion system, rebalance your gut wellbeing, and smolder off fat for good.

Flat Belly is about putting your hand solidly on the tiller and turning hard to starboard, directing your life far from the twin chunks of ice of corpulence and sickness and out beyond all detectable inhibitions water of a superior predetermination.